HEALTH CARE CAREERS IN **2** YEARS ™

JUMP-STARTING A CAREER IN

HOSPITALS & HOME HEALTH CARE

JERI FREEDMAN

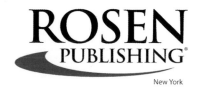

ROSEN
PUBLISHING®

New York

Published in 2014 by The Rosen Publishing Group, Inc.
29 East 21st Street, New York, NY 10010

Copyright © 2014 by The Rosen Publishing Group, Inc.

First Edition

Library of Congress Cataloging-in-Publication Data

Freedman, Jeri.
Jump-starting a career in hospitals & home health care/Jeri Freedman.
— First edition.
    pages cm. — (Health care careers in 2 years)
Audience: Grades 7-12.
Includes bibliographical references and index.
ISBN 978-1-4777-1696-0 (library binding)
1. Home health aides—Vocational guidance. 2. Nurses' aides—Vocational guidance. 3. Allied health personnel—Vocational guidance. I. Title.
RA645.3.F74 2014
610.73'7069--dc23

2013013959

Manufactured in Malaysia

CPSIA Compliance Information: Batch #W14YA: For further information, contact Rosen Publishing, New York, New York, at 1-800-237-9932.

CONTENTS

INTRODUCTION

The ambulance, sirens screaming, pulled up to the emergency entrance of the hospital. Emergency medical technicians (EMTs) jumped out and removed the accident victim, rolling him through the doors on a gurney to a cubicle in the emergency room. As medical staff examined the victim, a phlebotomist drew blood and sent it to the hospital lab to be tested. In the lab, a laboratory technician tested the blood, screening it for medically important elements and drugs.

Meanwhile, the admissions clerk spoke with the patient's family, getting information necessary to treat the patient. The patient was taken to the radiology department, where a radiological technician took scans of his body to provide physicians with the information they needed to operate. While the patient was in surgery, the social work assistant talked to the family. After surgery, she would help them arrange rehabilitation services for the patient when he left the hospital.

All of the people in this scenario are part of the team that makes it possible to treat people and save lives in a hospital—and they all have jobs that require two years or less of training. The hospital and home health care fields offer a number of opportunities for a challenging and fulfilling career—one that makes a difference in people's lives. Moreover, these fields have a strong and growing

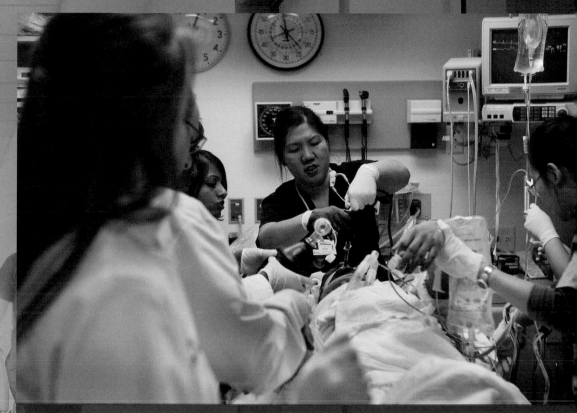

Staff in a hospital trauma center work to save a patient's life. Working in a hospital is challenging and can make a real difference in people's lives.

demand for employees. So, even in a stagnant economy, there are excellent prospects for finding a job. In addition to the large number of job opportunities, careers in the hospital and home health care fields provide the satisfaction of doing work that helps others. Job functions range from hands-on patient care to laboratory work to operating high-technology equipment.

The hospital and home health fields offer many jobs that don't require a four-year college degree. They provide excellent career opportunities with affordable training requirements. Some occupations provide on-the-job training; others require the completion of educational programs ranging from a few months to two years long. Some jobs require hands-on training and practice in areas such as drawing blood or using medical equipment. However, other jobs, including medical transcription and medical coding and billing, are suitable for online or distance education. Learning the course material and passing a certification test offered by the appropriate professional organization can provide the necessary job credentials without attending classes in person.

The following information covers the different types of jobs available in the hospital and home health care fields. It provides information on the educational and training requirements as well as the duties involved. It describes the steps you should follow in finding and applying for a job. Finally, it includes information on expanding your horizons in the field after you are employed.

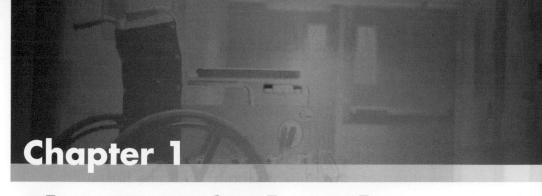

Chapter 1

The Hospital and Home Health Fields

One of the challenges faced by high school graduates who do not plan to go to college is finding a good job. The health care field offers opportunities for people with all levels of training and experience. Even entry-level jobs in this field can make a difference in people's lives, and these positions offer job security and, frequently, good benefits.

There are a large number of health care jobs—in both hospitals and private home health care organizations— that do not require advanced medical degrees from expensive universities. High school graduates can obtain many of these positions with on-the-job or a small amount of training. Some jobs require the completion of a training program that may range from a few months to two years in length.

In many cases, entry-level jobs can be the first step to a more advanced position in the health care field. Employees can advance through promotion as they gain more experience. Many people who start out in entry-level jobs choose to pursue more training while working and go on to obtain certifications or degrees.

In many cases, financial assistance for additional training is available through employers' tuition reimbursement
programs or government programs. Some hospitals
allow employees to participate in training programs that
they offer for free or at a reduced cost.

Many of the jobs described here require little previous
training and minimal coursework. Therefore, potential
employers often focus on personality traits as much as
education and experience when evaluating job candidates. For those seeking a career in a hospital or in home
health care, personal qualities may be as important as
training. Employees in this field work with people who
are unwell and, frequently, with family members who are
stressed. Employers are looking for people with traits such
as a pleasant personality, patience, attention to detail,
and problem-solving skills. Because health care is often
delivered by a team of professionals, the ability to work
well with others is also highly desired.

In the past few decades, changes in the population
have created a tremendous demand for health care workers. Because of this, jobs are likely to remain plentiful in
this field for a long time.

The Changing Health Care Industry

The nature of the health care industry in the United States
has changed significantly over the past fifty years. Until
the 1970s, most people covered by health insurance had
an indemnity plan. With this type of insurance plan,
patients could go to any health care provider or facility
they chose, and the insurance company paid for what-
ever services were provided. Decisions on treatment were

made strictly between the doctor and patient, with no input from the insurance company.

This form of insurance is rarely seen anymore. As health care costs started to increase significantly during the 1970s, insurance companies sought ways to control costs. They began asserting greater control over issues such as appropriate treatment for various conditions and the length of hospital stays. The efforts of health insurance companies to reduce the cost of health care have led to a greater reliance on non-physician personnel to treat patients. They have also led to shorter hospital stays and increased use of home health care.

Many activities that were once performed in hospitals are now performed at home by patients and their families with the assistance of home health care personnel. As a result, demand has increased for nurses, physician's assistants, medical assistants, personal care aides, and home health aides. This approach to providing medical treatment has resulted in many jobs that require two years or less of training. Therefore, the health care field is an excellent match for those seeking a career with good long-term prospects that does not require a four-year college degree.

Another change that has taken place is the aging of the population. The baby boomer generation consists of people born between the end of World War II and the early 1960s. This population explosion represented the largest number of people born in a single generation in U.S. history. Members of the baby boomer generation are now ages fifty to seventy. Because people usually have more health issues as they age, this large aging population is creating an increasing demand for health care and home

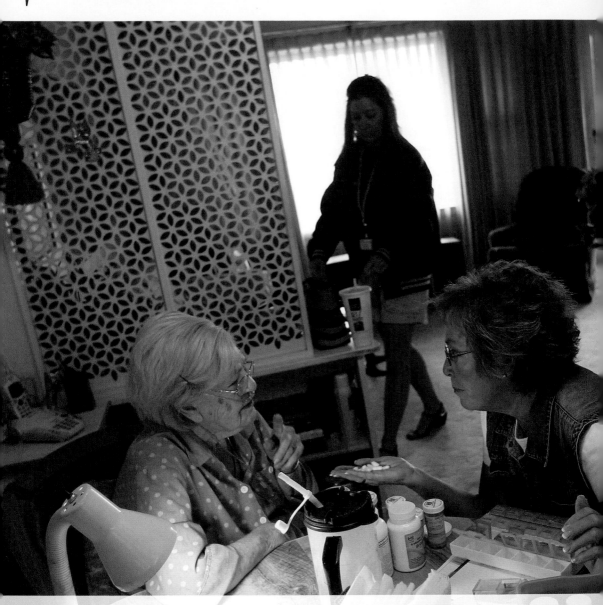

A nurse explains medication to an elderly patient during a home visit. People are living longer, creating a tremendous need for workers to care for the elderly.

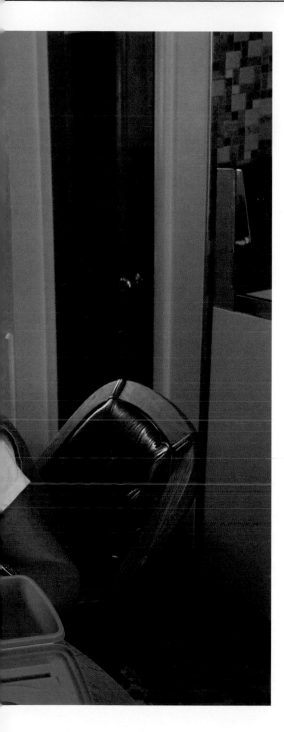

care services—and a corre-
sponding demand for
personnel to deliver these
services.

People are also living
longer. According to the
U.S. Social Security
Administration, in 1940, the
average life expectancy was
53.9 for a man and 60.6
for a woman. Today, the
average expected lifespan is
75.7 for a man and 80.8
for a woman, according to
the U.S. Census Bureau.
Increased lifespans have
also increased the demand
for health care services.

A third factor that has
affected the health care
system is the passage of the
Patient Protection and
Affordable Care Act of
2010. This act vastly
increased the number of
people covered by health
insurance. These previously
uninsured people are now
more likely to access health
care services. More people
accessing services means

more staff is required to serve them, both in hospitals and in their homes.

Hospitals and Related Facilities

The hospital field consists of general and specialty hospitals. General hospitals, as the name suggests, provide a wide range of services. These may include surgery, treatment for trauma from accidents, treatment for various diseases and injuries, delivering babies, and in some cases, mental health services.

Specialty hospitals handle only one type of problem. For example, mental health hospitals specialize in treating people with psychological problems. Rehabilitation hospitals help people recover physical functions after injury or surgery. There are facilities that specialize in treating cancer or in treating burn patients. Hospices are facilities that provide support and comfort for people who are dying.

Most patients stay in hospitals for relatively brief periods. However, after treatment some patients are not well enough to return home, but they are not sick enough to require a high level of skilled medical care. Such patients are often transferred to long-term-care facilities, where they receive supportive care and assistance until they are well enough to return home.

Most hospitals provide inpatient and outpatient services. Inpatient treatment requires a patient to check into a hospital and stay for one or more days. Inpatient hospital treatment is usually associated with surgery or serious illness. In these situations, patients may need to stay in the hospital until their physician decides that they are

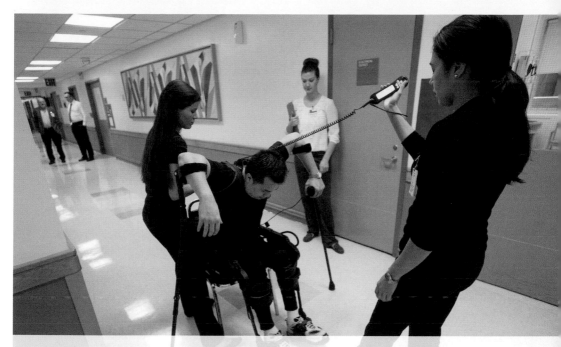

Hospital staff at Mount Sinai Medical Center in New York work with a patient to improve his mobility. A robotic exoskeleton helps the patient progress from sitting to standing.

sufficiently recovered to go home. Many specialty hospitals such as mental health or rehabilitation hospitals also provide inpatient treatment. With outpatient treatment, the patient comes to the hospital, receives treatment, and goes home again. Outpatient treatment may take the form of a one-time treatment, such as minor surgery, or it may require repeated visits over a period of weeks.

Working in a hospital can be rewarding because it can have a positive effect on people's lives. It can be interesting and exciting. However, working in a hospital

THE OUTLOOK FOR THE HOSPITAL AND HOME HEALTH CARE INDUSTRIES

Health care is one of the fasting-growing industries. According to the U.S. Bureau of Labor Statistics (BLS), the demand for health care staff is great and is expected to continue to grow well into the future. The BLS has projected that the demand for EMTs and paramedics will grow at the rate of 33 percent from 2010 through 2020. The demand for medical assistants is expected to increase by 31 percent. This is partly due to an increase in the number of patients that doctors see, which requires them to delegate more routine tasks to other staff members. The demand for nurse's aides, orderlies, and attendants is expected to grow by 20 percent. Because of the increase in the elderly population, long-term-care facilities will require more staff. The demand for medical records and information clerks is expected to increase by 21 percent, as the rising number of patients creates more health records and reimbursement claims. The demand for technicians and technologists in cardiovascular (heart and circulatory system) imaging and procedures is expected to increase by 29 percent. Radiographic technicians, who take X-rays and perform diagnostic imaging scans, will see demand increase by 28 percent. The demand for licensed practical and vocational nurses is expected to increase by 22 percent.

While large, all of these figures are dwarfed by the expected increase in demand for home health care personnel. The demand for home health aides is projected to grow by 69 percent, and the demand for personal care aides by 70 percent. Given the large projected increase in demand, careers in health care should provide considerable job security for a long time to come.

can also be stressful. One may have to deal with a large number of patients and tasks at the same time. Crises can occur unexpectedly, and one must pay careful attention to every task performed because mistakes can have serious consequences for a patient's health.

Home Health Careers

Home health care is the providing of personal care and health care in a person's own home rather than in a medical facility. Most home health care is provided by private companies. These companies range from small companies that serve a local area to large corporations with branches in multiple states. They employ staff such as home care or personal care aides, home health aides, and licensed practical nurses.

Home health care companies provide services to people who have recently had medical procedures in the hospital and need ongoing assistance or further procedures performed at home. They also provide services to the elderly and people with chronic medical problems who need assistance.

In addition to personal care and health care services, some home health companies provide sitter services. They provide a person to stay with an elderly, sick, or disabled person when his or her usual caregiver needs to be away from the home.

Working in home health care provides job security because there is a great demand for personnel in this field. The continued aging of the population is likely to create an even larger demand in the future. The

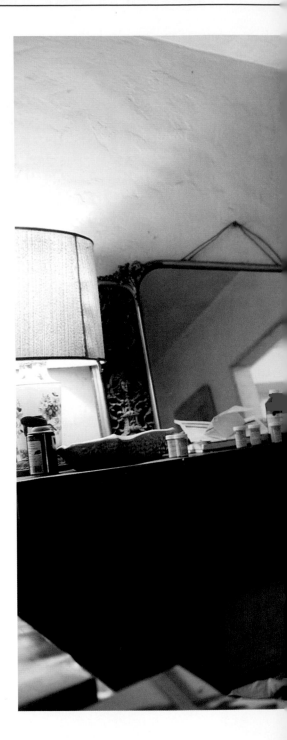

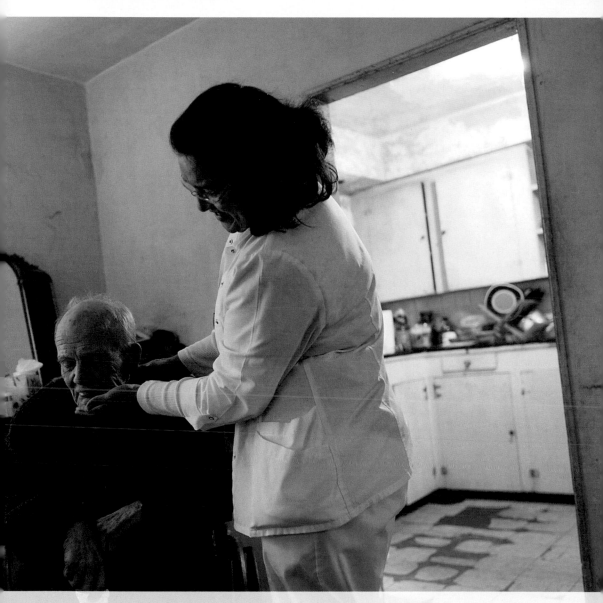

A home health aide assists an elderly patient with daily living tasks. Home health aides contribute greatly to the ability of elderly people to continue to live at home.

field can provide the personal satisfaction of helping people who need assistance and making a difference in people's lives. One drawback is that schedules can be difficult to predict and may require working outside of typical working hours. In addition, wages can be fairly low, especially in positions that require minimal education or credentials.

Education for Hospital and Health Care Careers

Many hospital and home health care careers require candidates to complete a training program ranging from several months to two years long. Courses for health care jobs are offered by technical and vocational schools, community colleges, specialized schools such as colleges of pharmacy or nursing, and traditional colleges.

In some cases, it is possible to complete coursework online. When passing a certification exam is the goal, the venue in which one takes a course is often less important than simply learning the material and passing the test. This is the case for areas such as medical transcription and coding.

If one takes the online approach to obtaining a two-year associate's degree, it is a good idea to check the U.S. Department of Education's online database of accredited schools (http://ope.ed.gov/accreditation/Search.aspx) to ensure that the school is accredited.

Certification and Licensing

Many jobs in the hospital and home health industry require certification or licensing. Certification is usually provided by industry organizations, such as the Association for Healthcare Documentation Integrity (AHDI), whereas licensing is provided by individual states. In both cases, applicants must meet the educational requirements and take a test demonstrating that they have mastered the subject matter in their field.

Certification and licensing are means of ensuring that workers who are responsible for the safety and health of people have mastered the skills of their profession. The courses one takes to prepare for a specific job typically provide the knowledge necessary to meet the requirements of licensing or certification in that field. In addition, special courses and books are often available to help one practice for these tests. Certification and licensing requirements for specific jobs are described later, in the sections on the different jobs.

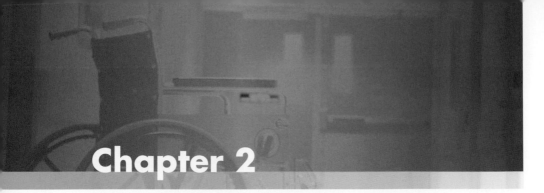

Chapter 2

Patient Care Jobs in Hospitals

Hospitals offer many jobs in patient care that are suitable for high school graduates. Some jobs require only a high school diploma, with the institution providing on-the-job training. Other jobs require a limited amount of additional training, ranging from a few weeks to two years.

Two types of patient care are provided in hospitals: scheduled, or elective, procedures and emergency procedures. An elective procedure is treatment that a patient chooses, or elects, to have done. In many cases, the treatment may be required to fix a problem—such as radiation treatment to treat cancer. However, it is still a procedure that the patient chooses to have and schedules in advance. Emergency care is provided in response to an unexpected trauma or accident, or a sudden serious illness. Most emergency care is provided through the emergency department. After emergency treatment, the patient may be sent home or admitted to the hospital for additional care.

The patient-care jobs described here cover the treatment of outpatients, who visit the hospital for treatment, and inpatients, who stay in the hospital for ongoing treatment or following surgery.

Emergency Medical Technician

One of the most exciting patient-care jobs is emergency medical technician (EMT). EMTs ride in ambulances and stabilize and transport patients who are extremely ill or are hurt in an accident or disaster. EMTs are trained in basic lifesaving techniques. They may administer medications under the direction of a physician with whom they are in contact. Because there are different levels of certification for EMTs, one can start with a minimal level of training and advance to higher levels by continuing one's education.

EMTs may work for private or hospital ambulance companies. The job can be physically and emotionally demanding. EMTs deal with people who have serious or life-threatening injuries and those who may be emotionally disturbed because of mental illness, substance abuse, or trauma. EMTs have to lift heavy people and equipment. In the case of disasters, they may have to work in chaotic and sometimes dangerous situations. However, this can be an exciting and meaningful career for someone who doesn't want to be restricted to a traditional nine-to-five job.

EMTs need certification and a license to work in their state. Requirements vary by state. There are three levels of certification for EMTs. To become an EMT-Basic, candidates typically take about one hundred hours of training. They learn basic lifesaving procedures, such as how to perform cardiopulmonary resuscitation (CPR), stop

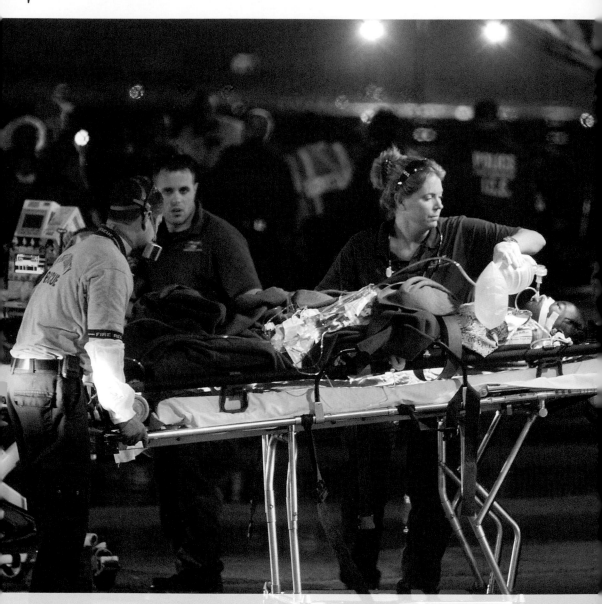

EMTs load an earthquake victim onto a gurney for transportation to a hospital. EMTs are often among the first responders in the event of a natural disaster.

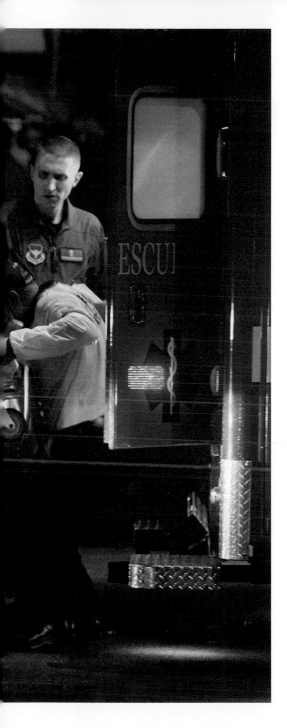

bleeding, stabilize fractures, treat drug overdoses, and deliver babies. This level of training can be completed in a few weeks or part-time over a few months. EMTs often staff ambulances, so they learn how to use basic emergency equipment and how to drive and maintain the ambulance.

By taking additional training to learn how to treat shock, insert breathing tubes in patients who are having difficulty breathing, and provide intravenous fluids, one can advance to EMT-Intermediate, also known as Advanced EMT. EMTs at this level typically complete about one thousand hours of training. Pay is generally higher at this level.

The most advanced EMT has the Paramedic certification. To qualify for this level, one must qualify as an EMT-Basic and Advanced EMT and complete additional training—about 1,300 hours total. Coursework

GAIN EXPERIENCE NOW

How do you make yourself stand out from other candidates for entry-level hospital jobs or training programs? One way is to gain some experience while still in high school. For example, a student can volunteer at a hospital, health clinic, or nursing home. Working with medical professionals in such an environment allows you to see if the health care field is appealing to you. It also provides the opportunity to see what kinds of work various employees perform.

Volunteering gives you the chance to develop the interpersonal skills necessary to successfully work with patients and staff in a medical environment. Beyond this, it allows you to make contacts with professionals in the industry who may be able to provide recommendations to potential employers and possibly provide assistance when the time comes to look for a job.

In some cases, it may be possible to obtain part-time or summer employment in a hospital. Working in any capacity in a medical facility can provide valuable experience to include on a résumé. For information on part-time and volunteer opportunities, contact the human resources departments of local hospitals and nursing homes. Major hospitals frequently have a volunteer coordinator who manages volunteers or even an entire volunteer department.

includes practical hands-on work in a hospital and an internship in the field. In addition to regular EMT functions, paramedics read diagnostic information from equipment such as electrocardiograph machines, which show how the heart is beating. They can administer medication ordered by a physician and use a device called a defibrillator to restart a person's heart.

EMT courses at all levels are offered at colleges and universities, community colleges, technical institutes, and other facilities that specialize in emergency training. Individual states have agencies with which EMTs must register or be licensed in order to work. Once a person has completed the requirements to become an EMT at any level, he or she can take an examination to become certified by the National Registry of Emergency Medical Technicians (NREMT). Some states require this certification for state licensure. EMTs are generally required to recertify every few years and take a certain number of continuing education courses to keep their skills current.

Registered Nurse

Nurses provide care to patients in hospitals according to the orders of a physician. They administer medications and treatments, draw blood, check vital signs, operate and monitor medical equipment, and ensure that patients' needs are met while they are in the hospital. They also teach patients how to manage their illnesses or injuries while they are in the hospital and after they go home. A registered nurse (RN) can work in a variety of hospital settings, including operating rooms, emergency rooms, intensive care, pediatrics, neonatal units, and many more.

Becoming a registered nurse requires obtaining at least an associate's degree from a technical school or community college and then passing the National Council Licensure Examination—Registered Nurse (NCLEX-RN) offered by the National Council of State Boards of Nursing. Candidates also need to pass the state board of nursing in the state where they wish to practice. For most registered nurse positions, however, hospitals prefer job candidates who have a four-year bachelor's degree in nursing. Therefore, registered nurses with associate's degrees are most likely to be hired for lower-level nursing positions. An option is to start in such a position and then continue one's education. There are also other types of nursing jobs available to those who have two years or less of training.

Licensed Practical Nurse

Licensed practical nurses (LPNs), sometimes called licensed vocational nurses (LVNs), provide hands-on care to patients who are disabled, ill, or injured. LPNs provide nursing services under the direction of a registered nurse. They help patients with tasks such as washing, eating, and dressing. They also take patients' vital signs, change dressings on wounds, assist physicians during patient exams, record patient information, and carry out administrative work. LPN education consists of a twelve- to eighteen-month training program. The program includes practical training in a hospital as well as coursework in anatomy and physiology, first aid, nursing procedures, and medication administration, among other topics. LPN programs are offered at technical schools, community

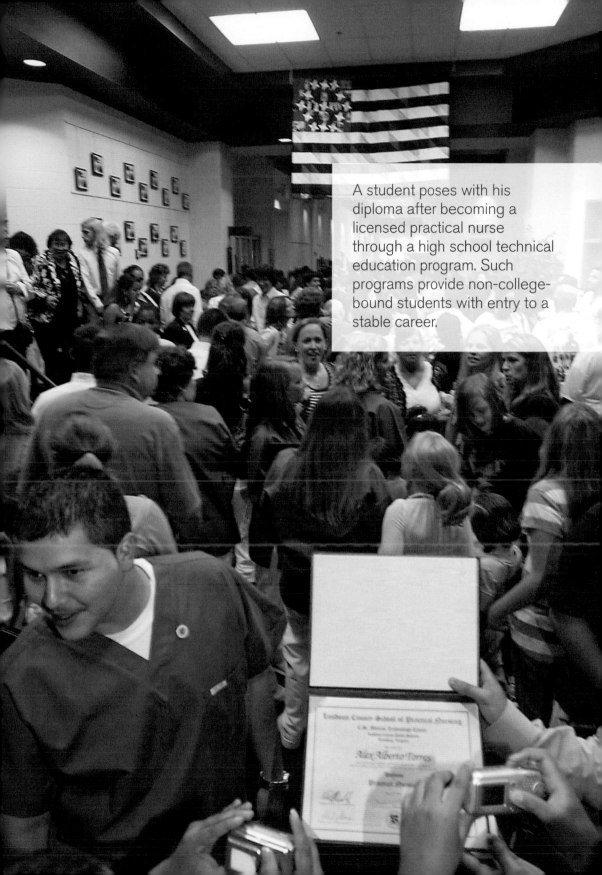

A student poses with his diploma after becoming a licensed practical nurse through a high school technical education program. Such programs provide non-college-bound students with entry to a stable career.

colleges, and hospitals. Students are awarded a certificate or a diploma upon completion. After obtaining a certificate or diploma, students take a licensing examination from the state licensing board in the state where they wish to practice.

Certified Nurse Assistant

Certified nurse assistants (CNAs) see to the physical needs of patients and assist registered nurses and licensed practical nurses. They help patients with daily activities such as eating, washing, and dressing. They work in hospitals, long-term-care facilities, and hospices. In long-term-care facilities, they often handle the bulk of patient-related activities.

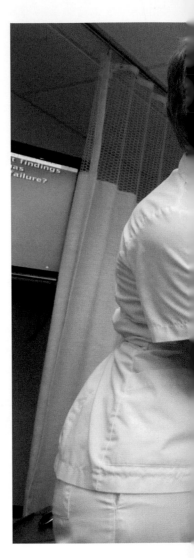

To become a CNA, a high school graduate undergoes 75 to 140 hours (2 to 8 weeks) of training. The training is provided at hospitals, technical schools, vocational schools, and health agencies. Most states require CNAs to be certified. Medical facilities that accept patients under Medicare and/or Medicaid must comply with the programs' guidelines, which require CNAs to undergo a competency evaluation within four months of being hired. To meet these requirements, CNAs take a written

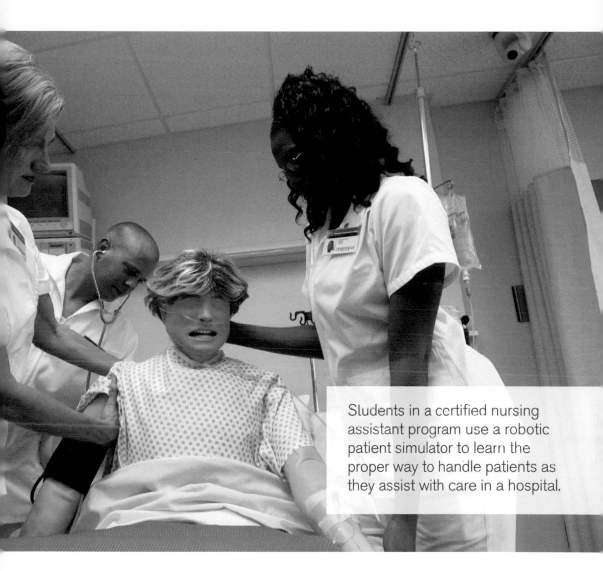

Students in a certified nursing assistant program use a robotic patient simulator to learn the proper way to handle patients as they assist with care in a hospital.

competency exam such as the National Nurse's Aide Assessment Program exam administered by the National Council of State Boards of Nursing.

Phlebotomist

Phlebotomists draw blood from patients, label the vials, and pass them on to the medical laboratory for evaluation. They usually work in hospital laboratories, where patients go to have blood drawn. By pursuing additional education, phlebotomists can become laboratory technicians. To become a phlebotomist, candidates must complete a course that takes a few weeks. Major aspects of training include learning to locate veins and insert a needle and draw blood without causing significant pain. Attention to detail is very important in this job, as mislabeling vials can have serious consequences.

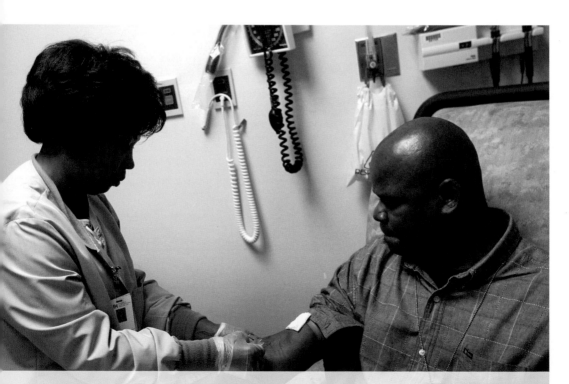

A phlebotomist draws blood from a patient for screening. Such screening is key to identifying early signs of disease or problems with internal organs.

Medical Assistant

Medical assistants perform a combination of clerical and medical work. Their responsibilities depend on training and experience. Their clerical duties include scheduling appointments, keeping records, coding medical records for billing purposes, and completing paperwork for prescriptions and lab tests. Their medical responsibilities may include setting up exam rooms; obtaining initial information from patients; and recording patients' height, weight, and vital signs, such as pulse and temperature. They may help patients get ready for an exam or treatment and assist the doctor

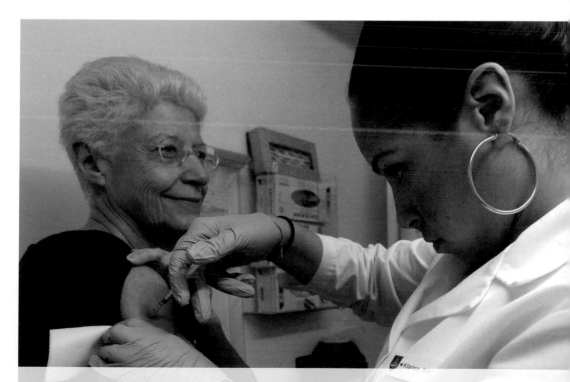

A medical assistant administers a flu shot to a patient. Medical assistants perform a combination of clinical and administrative functions, requiring good organizational and people skills.

during procedures. They also order and stock supplies, and they may clean or sterilize equipment. Medical assistants working for specialists may learn procedures specific to that medical specialty.

Medical assistants can undertake additional training to become physician's assistants who can perform more advanced medical procedures or move into supervisory administrative positions. Education for medical assistants consists of a one-year certificate program or a two-year associate's degree program. Accredited programs are offered at colleges and universities, community colleges, and technical schools. The American Association of Medical Assistants (AAMA) and American Medical Technologists (AMT) provide certification for medical assistants.

Orderly/Attendant

Orderlies, sometimes called medical attendants, perform routine tasks in a hospital under the direction of the medical or nursing staff. They transport patients to and from the operating room and other medical departments. They restock supplies, set up equipment, and assist nurses with patients as needed. This job requires only a high school diploma. Candidates for this position must be reliable and have good people skills.

Chapter 3

Technical Jobs in Hospitals

Diagnosing and treating patients requires a lot of machines and equipment. Hospitals require employees to operate and maintain this equipment. People in these positions have some contact with patients, although not as much as those who provide direct patient care. Technical jobs are also available running tests and analyzing samples in hospital laboratories.

Medical Equipment Technician/ Technologist

There are a variety of equipment technician and technologist jobs in hospitals. These jobs have several basic tasks in common. Medical equipment technologists are responsible for setting up and calibrating their equipment. They attach the equipment to patients and operate it. They check the equipment and perform basic maintenance on it.

There are two levels of technical equipment operators in hospitals: technicians and technologists. Technicians operate basic testing equipment. Technologists operate more advanced equipment and perform more complex procedures. Technician positions require a high school diploma and several months of on-the-job training. Technologist positions require completion of one to two years of formal training. Such training can be obtained at a community college, technical school, or hospital. Many colleges offer associate's degree programs that prepare technologists.

Technicians can advance to technologist positions by pursuing additional education, often on a part-time basis while working. Technologists can advance to supervisory positions.

The following are some types of medical equipment technicians and technologists:

- **Cardiovascular technician/technologist.** Cardiovascular technicians perform tests of heart function using an electrocardiograph (also called an EKG or ECG) machine. Cardiovascular technologists perform more advanced tests of heart function using equipment such as Holter monitors (portable devices worn by patients to record heart rhythm) and stress testing equipment. They use echocardiography machines, which use ultrasound waves to create images of the heart, and cardiac Doppler units, which use reflected sound waves to measure the output of blood from the heart.

- **Electroencephalographic technologist.** Electroencephalographic (EEG) technologists

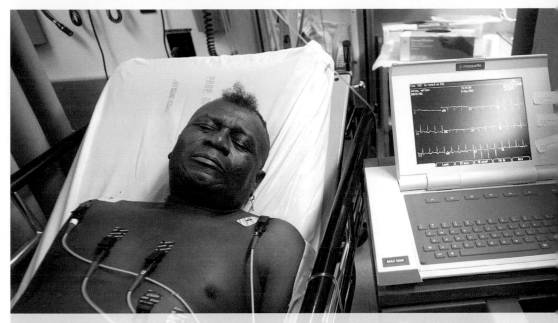

A patient undergoes an electrocardiogram in a hospital emergency room. Such tests can be critical in establishing if a patient is having a life-threatening problem, such as a heart attack.

operate the machine that analyzes brain waves, indicating normal and abnormal brain activity. High school graduates can either complete a one-year on-the-job training program or take a one- or two-year training program at a community college, technical school, or traditional college.

- **Pulmonary function technologist.** These technologists administer tests of breathing and lung function. They operate equipment used for exercise tolerance, sleep studies, and measuring oxygen and carbon dioxide in the blood. At the

LAYING THE GROUNDWORK

If you are interested in pursuing a career in a hospital, take as many science courses as possible. Chemistry and biology courses are particularly useful for understanding the material in future training programs and on the job. For those interested in a medical imaging or equipment technologist job, a course in physics can also be useful.

If you think there is a high probability that you will enter the workforce rather than go directly to college after completing high school, consider pursuing a program in career and technical education (CTE). Some high schools offer a program in health science, which can help one prepare to work in patient care. Many offer programs that provide training in science and technology skills, which can help one prepare for a job in technical equipment operation or laboratory work. Many offer clerical skills training. This kind of training can be valuable when pursuing a job as a medical assistant or applying for an administrative position in a hospital.

It is also necessary to learn to communicate well. Medical team members must frequently talk with physicians, other staff members, and patients, and document information in writing. Learn the rules of English grammar and composition and how to communicate ideas clearly. If your school offers computer technology classes, take them, since computers are used throughout medicine today. For the same reason, if your school offers a typing or keyboarding course, taking it can make your life easier in the future.

entry level, pulmonary function technologists may have a high school diploma and be trained on the job by a hospital. An associate's degree is generally preferred, however. People in this position can advance to higher levels of responsibility by obtaining a bachelor's degree.

- **Radiation therapist.** Radiation therapists operate equipment that is used to administer radiation treatment to cancer patients. They prepare patients for treatment, program the equipment delivering the radiation to the patient, and keep treatment records. Candidates can qualify for this position by taking a one- or two-year certificate program or obtaining a two-year associate's degree. Those who wish to move on to a supervisory position can pursue additional education and obtain a bachelor's degree.

Medical equipment technologists can obtain certification through professional organizations such as Cardiovascular Credentialing International (CCI), American Board of Registration for Electroencephalographic and Evoked Potential Technologists (ABRET), and others.

Imaging Technologists

Advanced imaging equipment has become a major tool in diagnosing patients. This equipment allows physicians to view the interior of a patient's body. Operating such equipment can provide an excellent career for those who are technically inclined.

There are a number of different medical imaging careers. Radiologic technologists, also called radiographers, use X-ray machines and other radiological equipment to take pictures, called radiographs, of the inside of people's bodies. Magnetic resonance imaging (MRI) technologists operate MRI equipment, which uses powerful electromagnets to take images of the inside of the body. Computed tomography (CT) scanning technologists operate computed tomography equipment. CT scanning uses computer processing to combine a series of X-rays, creating cross-sectional images of tissues inside the body.

Imaging technologists explain the procedure to patients, position patients for their scans, and operate the equipment to perform the scans. A two-year training program is required to become an imaging technologist. Many such programs are certificate programs offered through hospitals. They require a high school diploma

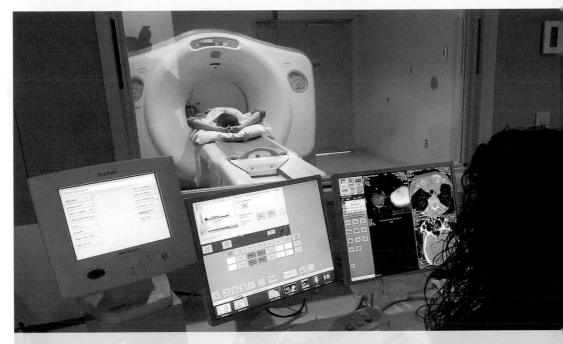

An imaging technician takes a CT scan of a patient. Such high-tech scanning equipment allows physicians to see problems inside patients' bodies.

for admission. Another option is an associate's degree program, typically offered by technical schools and community colleges. Upon completion of training, students must get certification from the American Registry of Radiologic Technologists (ARRT).

Sonographer

Sonographers use ultrasound equipment to take images of the inside of the body. Ultrasound equipment uses high-frequency sound waves to create images of structures inside the body. It is commonly used for imaging the brain, heart, abdomen, and blood vessels. It is also used to take images of fetuses in pregnant women. Sonographers position patients, apply gel to the skin, and run a handheld device over the area being scanned, adjusting the equipment to obtain a clear image. They also record the results of the scan.

Typically, sonographers complete an associate's degree program. To become certified, they can take an exam offered by the Society of Diagnostic Medical Sonography (SDMS).

Clinical Laboratory Technician

During diagnosis and treatment, physicians order many tests. These tests may be simple or complex. Clinical laboratory technicians, also called clinical laboratory assistants, perform the simpler tests, such as blood tests. They also prepare tissue samples for examination and carry out other routine laboratory procedures. Their supervisors are clinical laboratory technologists, who perform more advanced procedures.

Becoming a clinical laboratory technician requires an associate's degree. Clinical laboratory technicians can obtain certification from a variety of organizations, including the Board of Certification of the American Society for Clinical Pathology (ASCP) and the National Accrediting Agency for Clinical Laboratory Sciences (NAACLS), among others. Clinical laboratory technicians can go on to obtain a bachelor's degree and become clinical

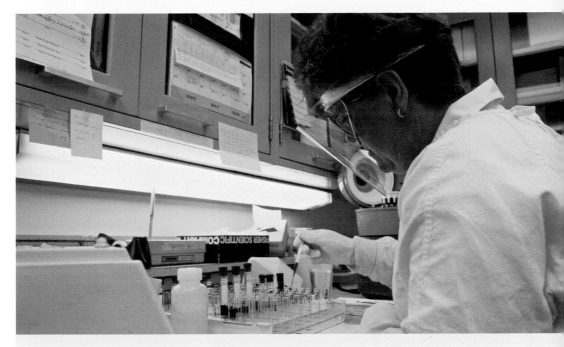

A clinical laboratory technician tests patients' blood. Such tests aid in identifying infections; thyroid, kidney, and liver diseases; AIDS; cancer; and many other disorders.

laboratory technologists and ultimately move on to supervisory positions.

Pharmacy Technician

Pharmacy technicians, sometimes called pharmacy assistants, prepare and distribute medications under the direction of the hospital pharmacist. They also restock pharmacy supplies. They field phone calls from nurses and

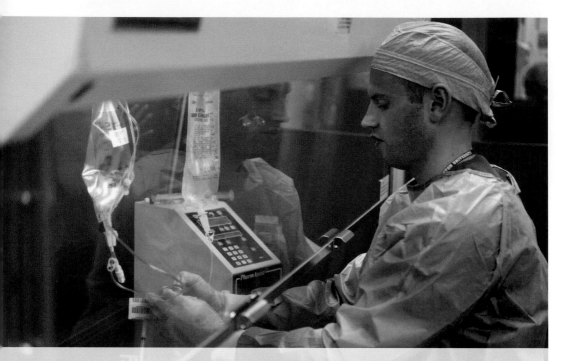

A pharmacy technician preloads doses of medicines from a bulk container into small syringes. Hospital nurses will use the syringes to administer medication to patients.

doctors who are ordering medications. They enter prescription information in the computer system and fill out forms to send to physicians when necessary. They also deliver medications to the areas of the hospital where patients are receiving treatment.

This job requires only a high school diploma. A few states require pharmacy technicians to be certified, which requires taking a pharmacy technician course online or at a college and then passing a test. Advancement in this field comes from pursuing further education to become a pharmacist.

Chapter 4

Nonclinical Jobs That Help Patients

There are many professionals working in hospitals who do not provide direct medical treatment or testing to patients. Although they have nonclinical roles, sometimes working in offices behind the scenes, these employees are important in making sure patients receive excellent care and the hospital functions smoothly. Such professionals include hospital administrators, medical records transcriptionists, social service aides, and interpreters.

Interpreter

Many hospitals employ interpreters today. The growing number of immigrants has created a great need for medical interpreters to communicate information between patients and medical staff. They work in the emergency room and in the hospital wards, obtaining consent from and explaining procedures to patients. They also assist hospital social services staff in arranging home health, nursing home, or other services for patients who don't speak English and are being discharged from the hospital.

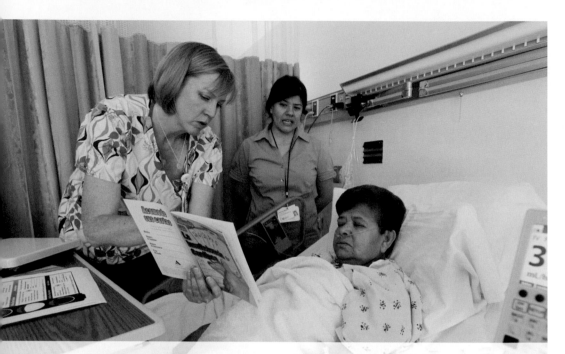

A hospital interpreter explains medical procedures and treatments in a patient's native language. Her work is key in avoiding misunderstanding and ensuring proper treatment.

People who are native or fluent speakers of a language other than English and who also have good English skills are in demand for this position. Languages in demand vary according to the ethnic mix of the area in which a facility is located. Interpreters are required for most common European languages, including eastern European ones. Languages often in high demand in urban areas include Spanish, Arabic, and Asian languages such as Chinese.

The only educational requirement in most cases is a high school diploma and fluency in at least one language other than English. Taking a course in medical terminology online or at a community college can be helpful. Skilled interpreters can also become medical translators, translating medical documents from English to other languages.

Social Service Aide

Social service aides help patients access necessary home health, community, and government resources and arrange services for them. They coordinate the transfer of hospital patients to "step-down," or transitional, facilities such as rehabilitation centers for those who are not ready to return home, or to hospice facilities for those with terminal illnesses. They also arrange home health care for patients being discharged from the hospital. They may help patients fill out forms to obtain follow-up resources from government programs such as Medicare and Medicaid. In addition, they provide information on community resources and assist the hospital social worker with other tasks.

This job usually requires only a high school diploma. Since many patients are not fluent in English, this is a good area for those just out of high school who are bilingual. Clerical skills and volunteer experience are also helpful. Taking sociology and psychology courses in high school, online, or at a community college enhances a candidate's chances of landing this job. People in this position may later pursue additional education to obtain a bachelor's degree to become social workers.

HOW TO GET HELP PAYING FOR YOUR EDUCATION

There are a variety of ways to get assistance in paying for health care training and education. Many technical schools and colleges have a financial aid department that helps students apply for financial aid. Some aid is available in the form of student loans. These loans are provided under government guidelines and have low interest rates. However, they must be repaid after graduation.

Some schools offer work-study programs, in which a student performs paid part-time work for the school. The Health Resources and Services Administration (HRSA), which is part of the U.S. Department of Health and Human Services, offers grants for low-income students who wish to study nursing, including those pursuing two-year associate's degrees. The funds are provided to schools, which choose the recipients. Check with the financial aid office at the schools you are considering, or visit the HRSA Web site (http://www.hrsa.gov/loanscholarships/scholarships/disadvantaged.html). Some states also offer grants for nursing students. Check with the state department of public health to see if any grants are available.

The U.S. Federal Supplemental Education Opportunity Grant program provides funds

to low-income students for education. Contact your school guidance counselor for information, or visit http://www2.ed.gov/ programs/fseog.

In addition, there are programs available to help fund the education of children of military veterans as well as the education of veterans themselves. Veterans and children of veterans should check with the Veterans Administration (http://www.gibill. va.gov) to see what educational financing programs they are eligible for.

Medical Records Transcriptionist/Clerk

Medical transcriptionists type up information from physicians describing the diagnosis and treatment of patients. Medical records clerks maintain and distribute information from patients' records. These jobs require knowledge of medical terminology and the ability to type and use a computer.

Candidates can train by taking an online or in-person course in medical transcription and medical records. The Association for Healthcare Documentation Integrity (AHDI) provides certification tests for medical transcriptionists; this can aid in obtaining a job. Medical records clerks and transcriptionists can move into supervisory positions in their departments or into other medical administrative positions.

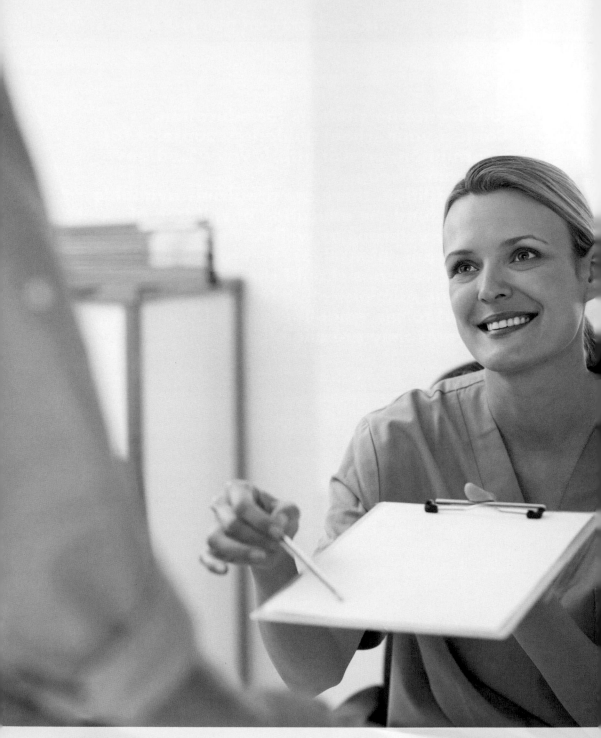

Medical records clerks maintain documentation of patients' health data and treatment information. Accurate information can be vital for present and future treatment of the patient.

Administrative Jobs

Hospitals require specialized clerical staff such as admitting clerks, medical receptionists, and schedulers. They also have many medical billing clerks, who code and submit information to insurance companies and government reimbursement programs to obtain payment for services.

With the exception of medical billing clerks, there are no particular educational requirements for these positions. However, taking courses in areas such as keyboarding, word processing, and spreadsheet programs enhances one's chances of landing an administrative job. Taking a course in medical terminology can be useful, too. Medical billing requires knowledge of the coding system used for billing purposes. Therefore, it is desirable to take a medical billing course online or at a community college.

Those in administrative positions can be promoted to supervisory positions and ultimately to a department manager position. Pursuing college-level business or hospital management courses can help in obtaining the position of manager.

Chapter 5

Jobs in Home Health Care

H ome health care is one of the fastest-growing segments of the health care industry. Because of the emphasis on getting patients out of hospitals faster and the aging of the population, there has been a continuous increase in the demand for home health care workers. This trend is expected to continue in the future.

Most home health care services are offered by private businesses. They provide aides to those who need personal and health care at home. Most aides visit a number of patients from one to several times a week. These jobs usually require a driver's license and a vehicle so that aides can drive themselves to patients' homes. They also require patience, reliability, and the ability to be courteous and pleasant even when patients are irritable, frustrated, or confused.

Personal Care Aide

Personal care aides provide assistance with tasks such as bathing, eating, dressing, and similar activities. They may cook food, perform housecleaning chores, and run errands. They may also drive patients to places such as the doctor's office.

In addition to providing services during scheduled visits, some home health care companies provide "sitter" services on an hourly basis. The personal care aide may stay with an individual for a number of hours or even a whole day while the person's usual caregiver is away from home. Personal care aides may work for a home health company on a full-time or part-time basis, so the job offers flexibility.

A job as a personal care aide does not require any special education. A pleasant personality, patience, and reliability are key factors in succeeding in this job. Because it is possible to arrange flexible hours, this is a good job for those who wish to continue their education part-time while working.

Certified Home Health Aide

Certified home health aides visit patients in their homes. In addition, they set up equipment and train patients and caretakers in the use of it. They take patients' vital signs, record information about their symptoms, and report any issues with a patient's mental, physical, or emotional condition to the care supervisor (usually a nurse in charge of the patient's case). They may also assist patients with personal care tasks.

Certified home health aides must complete a certified nursing assistant or home health aide course. These courses take place over several weeks and are available at technical schools, hospitals, and community colleges.

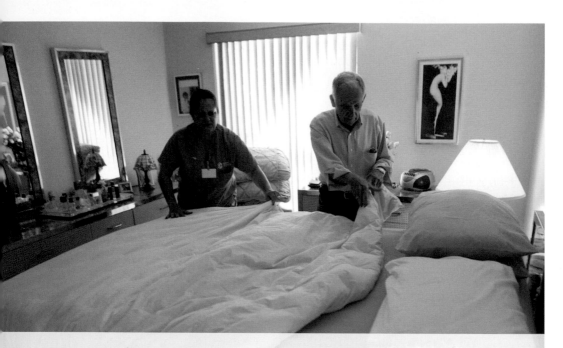

A home health aide assists with household tasks. Such aides can make a tremendous difference in the quality of life of elderly and disabled people.

Following completion of the course, students must pass a competency exam to demonstrate that they have mastered the material. One such exam is the National Nurse Aide Assessment Program (NNAAP) administered by the National Council of State Boards of Nursing (NCSBN).

Licensed Visiting Nurse

Home health care services have nurses who visit patients initially to evaluate their needs. They then visit periodically to check on the patients' health. Visiting nurses change dressings on wounds, administer medication, and take

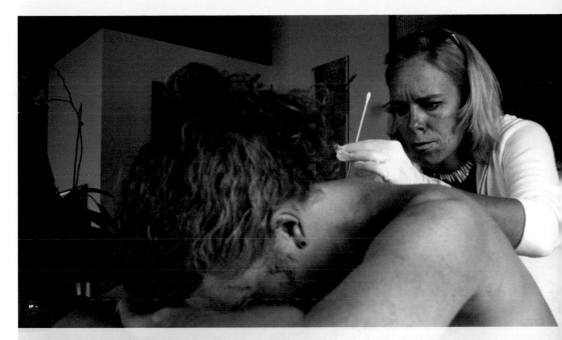

A licensed visiting nurse checks an incision in a patient recovering from surgery at home. LVNs play a vital role in ensuring that patients at home heal properly without problems.

patients' vital signs. They adjust equipment that dispenses medication, answer patients' questions, and arrange additional services if necessary.

Many home health care companies hire licensed practical or vocational nurses for these positions. One can become a licensed practical or vocational nurse by completing a one- or two-year course at a hospital, technical school, or community college and then taking a licensing test from the state board of nursing in the state where one wishes to practice.

Visiting nurses can move into administrative positions in home health care companies, such as patient care

COMMUNICATION SKILLS

The ability to communicate clearly is of great importance in health care. One must learn to listen carefully and convey information clearly and correctly because people's health and safety depend on it.

The first step in communication is making sure you understand information correctly. When someone is speaking to you, whether it is a staff member or patient, focus directly on that person and his or her words. Confirm that you understand what the speaker is saying by repeating what he or she said. That way, you are certain to get the meaning correct.

When conveying information to staff members or patients, first organize what you want to say so that the information is clear, easy to understand, and complete. Make sure the language you use is appropriate for the person to whom you are speaking. When speaking to staff, use appropriate medical terminology and grammatical English so that your meaning is clear. When speaking to patients or their family members, avoid using complicated medical terms. Instead explain information in a way that a layperson will understand.

Always speak in a respectful manner. Do not talk down to patients or their families. Be sensitive to the fact that they may be under stress and have difficulty absorbing information. If instructions are involved, ask them to repeat their understanding of what they are required to do so that you know they have understood the information correctly.

Learn to write clearly and correctly so that there is no confusion about the information you are recording. Make sure you write legibly for the same reason. Always read over what you have written, whether you are writing by hand on a chart or recording information on a computer. It's common to accidentally omit words or write the wrong word. In health care, misrecording information can have serious consequences, so be sure to double-check all your work. Because communication is critical in the medical field, how you present yourself orally and in writing when applying for a job will affect your chances of being hired.

recruiter and scheduler, or benefits coordinator. Patient care recruiters and schedulers recruit, train, and schedule home health personnel. Benefits coordinators meet with patients, families, and caregivers to design a plan for each patient, identifying which home health services are required. They then verify that the services are covered by the patient's insurance or government programs, such as Medicare or Medicaid, and arrange for the required personnel to attend the patient in his or her home.

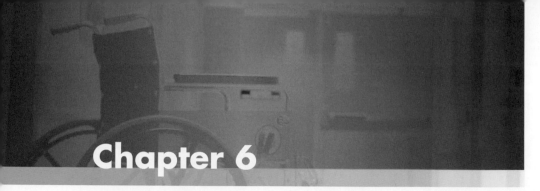

Chapter 6

Landing a Job and Advancing in One's Career

nce you have decided what job to pursue, the next step is to locate positions and land one. This section covers how to find job openings and obtain an interview. It also describes how you can progress in your career toward more advanced opportunities.

Locating Potential Jobs

The most obvious way to locate potential jobs is through online job postings. For example, sites such as CareerBuilder.com and Monster.com provide lists of health care jobs by type and location. Because of the shortage of personnel in areas such as home health care, responding to such ads may result in a job. However, large numbers of people usually respond to every ad on popular job sites. Therefore, competition can be much greater than with other approaches to job hunting. There are several other ways to locate potential jobs in the hospital and home health care fields.

If you take any courses to prepare for a health care career, your school may offer job placement resources. Technical schools and colleges usually have a job placement office that assists students in locating jobs. This office may also provide assistance with job-hunting skills and preparing résumés.

Job fairs are sometimes held at schools or in the community at large. At these fairs, representatives of companies talk to candidates about available jobs and collect résumés.

There is a lot of turnover in health care support jobs, and the high demand for services creates a continuous need for additional staff. Therefore, hospitals and home health care agencies frequently develop openings for personnel. Many institutions accept applications for positions in person at their human resources (HR) departments. An effective strategy is to research a list of hospitals and home health care agencies in your area. Then you can call these organizations and see if positions are available. Contact the HR department for information on job openings. In some cases, health facilities and home health care companies accept applications from candidates on an ongoing basis for home health aide and medical support jobs. Therefore, even if a job isn't immediately available, you may get a call when a position opens up.

Temporary help agencies are another source of jobs. Some companies specialize in supplying personnel to medical facilities on an as-needed basis. You can look for and contact temporary employment agencies in your area that specialize in health care.

In addition, many hospitals and health care organizations advertise job openings on their own Web sites and on

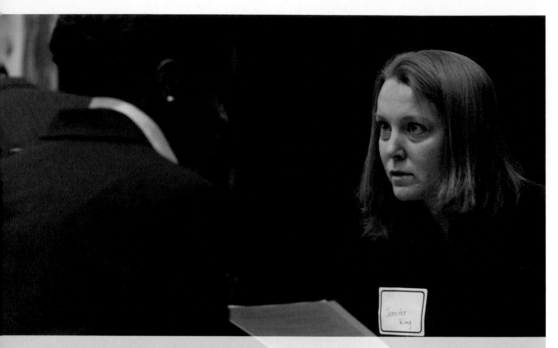

An applicant talks to a medical recruiter. The demand for personnel in health care is greater than in many other fields, providing numerous options for qualified job seekers.

general job-hunting Web sites. Once you have researched a list of home health care companies or hospitals in your area, check those organizations' Web sites. Many sites have links labeled "Jobs" or "Careers" that list open positions.

Also, check the Web site of the professional organization that covers your occupation. Often professional organizations maintain lists of job openings for members on their Web sites. Some organizations also have information on internship positions for students in the profession.

Internships are unpaid positions that give students a chance to learn about a job while still in school.

Preparing Your Résumé

When applying for a job, it is necessary to supply potential employers with a résumé. A résumé is a document that lists your skills, experience, and training. The purpose of the résumé is to convince the organization to give you an interview. Therefore, your résumé should focus on skills that apply specifically to the job for which you are applying.

The résumé should use a simple, easy-to-follow format. Start with personal information such as name, address, phone number, and e-mail address. Next, list any jobs you have held, with the most recent first. If they are relevant, you can list any part-time and summer jobs you have had, and include volunteer work you have performed at health care facilities or nursing homes.

Next, list your education. Include any certificate or degree course work you have completed, and list any certifications or other credentials you have obtained. Candidates who are applying for a job directly out of high school without completing a formal training program face a challenge. They must demonstrate to potential employers that they can handle the job, even though they do not have much previous work experience. To reassure potential employers that you have the knowledge to do the job, list relevant courses that you have taken in high school, such as biology, chemistry, physics, and computer technology, as well as any vocational courses that provide medical, technical, or administrative skills.

PARTICIPATING IN PROFESSIONAL ORGANIZATIONS

Most professions in the hospital and home health care fields have a professional organization. There are professional organizations for nurses, medical assistants, and nurse's aides; clinical laboratory technicians and technologists; EMTs; administrative personnel; and many other health professionals. Participating in professional organizations is important when looking for a job as well as after a person has landed one. Many organizations maintain lists of job openings on their Web sites, which are available to members looking for work. Professional organizations offer many benefits beyond this, however. Participating in meetings and conferences and reading an organization's publications can help members stay current on developments in their field and make them aware of new techniques and technologies.

Participation also provides the opportunity to network with other members. These contacts may be able to provide advice or help in dealing with issues when they arise. Participating in a professional organization also gives one the opportunity to affect one's profession. Members can work to improve working conditions or help create standards for the field, for example.

If you speak a language other than English, list this as well. With the many non-English-speaking patients in the health care system, being bilingual can be a major advantage when applying for a job.

Be sure to proofread your résumé—or better yet, have someone else read it. Those working in the health care field must be conscientious and detail-oriented because people's lives and health are at stake. You do not want to give potential employers the impression that you are careless or sloppy by sending them a résumé with mistakes in it.

Interviewing for a Health Care Job

The interview provides you with the opportunity to convince a prospective employer to hire you. Before you go to an interview, research the organization on the Internet so that you can show you understand what the organization does and what the job requires.

How you present yourself has a significant effect on your chances of being hired. Dress in neat, clean, professional-looking clothing and be well groomed. Speak respectfully, using correct grammar. If you are asked about experience or skills that you don't have, explain how your education or background equips you to learn those skills. It's not unusual for interviewers to ask questions designed to see how applicants react under stress or analyze problems. Realize that what the interviewer really wants to know is how you would approach solving a problem, rather than whether you can come up with a particular solution. Show how you would break the problem down to solve it, or show that you know when

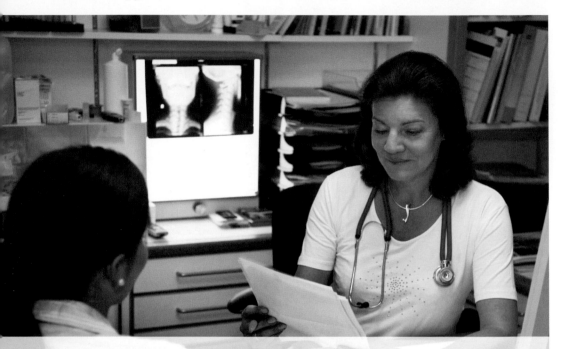

Hospitals look for applicants who act mature and professional, so personal presentation and attitude are important when interviewing for a job, especially if one is young.

you should contact a superior for assistance. It's a good idea to practice answering difficult but predictable questions such as "Tell me about yourself" or "What are your weaknesses?" That way, you can answer fluently when asked.

You are likely to be asked whether you will be responsible, show up on time, and perform tasks without supervision. It's a good idea to prepare examples of activities you have carried out responsibly, especially ones that involved looking after others. Even if you are not asked specifically, show that you understand the need for responsibility and reliability. Finally, be sure to be polite to everyone you meet because interviewers evaluate applicants' people skills as well as their practical skills, especially in a people-focused field such as health care.

Being Professional

Workers in the health care field are constantly in contact with members of the public and professionals such as physicians. Therefore, looking and sounding professional is important both when applying for a job and once you have obtained one.

When interviewing for a job, ensure that your clothing is appropriate for a professional: a suit or slacks, shirt, and jacket for men and a skirt suit, business-appropriate dress, or pantsuit for women. Your shoes should be polished and your hair cut. It is not appropriate to wear piercings or loud makeup or jewelry. Don't make the mistake of thinking that because workers wear a uniform, scrubs, or a lab coat on the job, casual clothing is appropriate for an interview. Being properly dressed makes interviewers see you as someone who knows how to be professional and has potential. The same applies to your appearance once you have obtained a position. If your job does not require wearing a uniform or scrubs, always dress neatly in business-appropriate clothing. Managers are more likely to promote those whom they view as professional.

Advanced Careers

When choosing a career, it's natural to wonder what kind of long-term prospects the field provides. This section covers some of the higher positions that one can attain after gaining significant experience and/or pursuing additional education. There are many opportunities to continue one's education part-time while working in the health care field, and employers often offer their workers tuition reimbursement for doing so. In some cases, hospitals may even offer employees free training or reduced fees for courses provided by the facility.

Those who start out as licensed practical nurses can expand their education by obtaining a bachelor's degree in nursing and becoming a registered nurse, or RN. RNs can rise to a managerial level, becoming nursing supervisors or nursing administrators. They can also pursue further education to become a nurse-midwife, who delivers

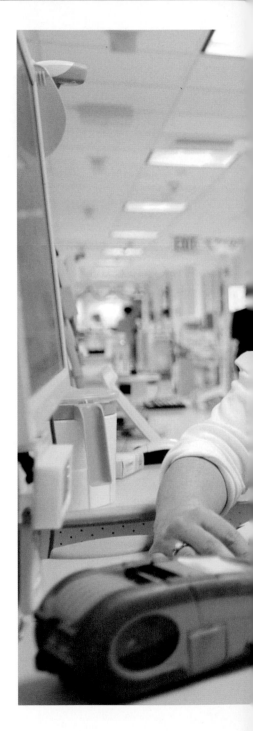

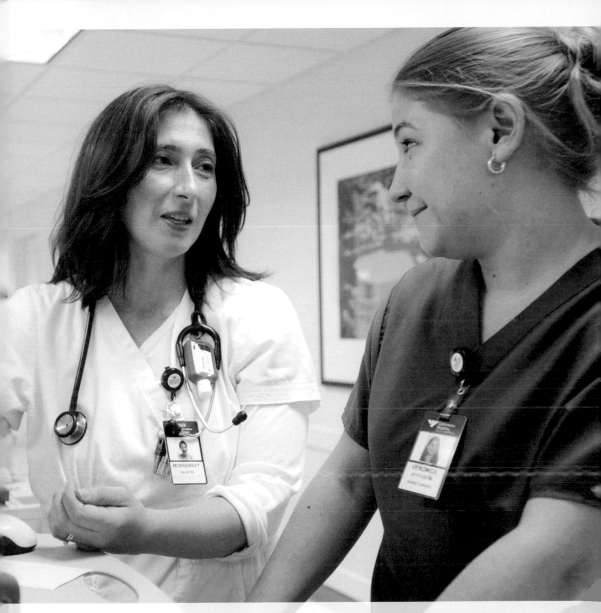

A registered nurse works with a young colleague. By gaining experience and pursuing additional education, a young nurse can advance to positions of greater authority and responsibility.

babies; a nurse-anesthetist, who administers anesthesia during surgery; or a nurse practitioner or physician's assistant, who diagnoses and treats patients under the direction of a physician. Medical assistants can pursue additional education to become physician's assistants.

Some home health aides eventually become freelancers after they have acquired sufficient experience. They offer their services directly to people who need assistance by advertising in newspapers and senior publications and through online Web sites. By providing their services directly and not through a home health company, they keep all of the hourly fees they charge. While freelancers or independent contractors can make more money, they receive no company-supplied benefits, and so they must pay for expenses like health insurance. They also need to do their own marketing to find customers.

Another track for advancement is moving into management. Those in administrative positions can move up to the level of shift supervisor and department supervisor. By pursuing additional education in hospital or health care management, they can eventually move into higher management.

Those who work in technical positions can move into supervisory or lab management positions. They can also move into the medical products industry, working in research laboratories, product development, or product sales. Pursuing a bachelor's degree or graduate degree enhances their job opportunities in such companies.

The careers described here offer entry to a field that can provide a stable and fulfilling job in the present, as well as lifelong career opportunities.

GLOSSARY

accredited Officially recognized as maintaining appropriate educational standards, especially for preparing graduates for professional practice.

administrative Relating to the running of an organization or business.

calibrate To check, adjust, or standardize a measuring instrument.

cardiopulmonary resuscitation (CPR) An emergency procedure designed to revive a person whose heart and breathing have stopped by compressing the chest and forcing air into the lungs.

cardiovascular Relating to the heart and circulatory system.

chronic Continuing for a long time or frequently recurring.

competency The state of having the necessary abilities or skills.

defibrillator A device that delivers an electric current to the heart to restore normal heart rhythms.

echocardiography The use of ultrasound to examine the structure and functioning of the heart and diagnose abnormalities.

electrocardiography The recording of electrical activity in the heart prior to each heartbeat and the study and interpretation of the recordings.

inpatient A patient who stays in a hospital or other health facility while receiving treatment.

intravenous Inserted directly into a vein.

magnetic resonance imaging (MRI) A technology that uses large magnets and electric current to create images of the inside of the body.

medical transcriptionist A professional who prepares a written record of patient medical reports dictated by a physician.

neonatal Of or relating to newborn infants, especially to their care during the first few weeks of life.

nonclinical Not involving direct observation and treatment of patients.

outpatient A patient who visits a hospital or other health facility for diagnosis or treatment but does not stay overnight.

stress test The process of measuring the performance of a person's heart during physical exertion by recording the person's heart rate, blood pressure, oxygen intake, and other factors.

vital signs Basic measurements of body function, such as temperature, pulse, respiration, and blood pressure.

American Association of Medical Assistants (AAMA)
20 N. Wacker Drive, Suite 1575
Chicago, IL 60606
(312) 899-1500
Web site: http://www.aama-ntl.org
AAMA provides certification for medical assistants, local
chapters where they can meet and discuss issues, and
other professional resources.

American Board of Registration for Electroencephalographic
and Evoked Potential Technologists (ABRET)
2509 West Iles Avenue, Suite 102
Springfield, IL 62704
(217) 726-7980
Web site: http://abret.org
ABRET focuses on the competency and evaluation of
technologists serving the neurology community and its
patients. It provides credentials in the field of neurodi-
agnostics, including those for EEG, evoked potential,
neurophysiologic intraoperative monitoring, and long-
term monitoring technologists.

American Medical Technologists (AMT)
10700 West Higgins, Suite 150
Rosemont, IL 60018
(800) 275-1258
Web site: http://www.americanmedtech.org
This organization provides certification of medical technologists. It offers a variety of resources for students, including
student memberships and scholarships and awards.

American Registry of Radiological Technicians (ARRT)
1255 Northland Drive
St. Paul, MN 55120
(651) 687-0048
Web site: https://www.arrt.org
ARRT provides certification for radiological technicians. Its
    Web site includes information for students on
    certification.

American Society of Clinical Pathology (ASCP)
33 West Monroe Street, Suite 1600
Chicago, IL 60603
(800) 267-2727
Web site: http://www.ascp.org
ASCP is a professional membership organization for
    pathologists and laboratory professionals. Its mission is
    to provide excellence in education, certification, and
    advocacy on behalf of patients, pathologists, and
    laboratory professionals across the globe. Its Web site
    provides resources for students, including publications
    and scholarships.

Association for Healthcare Documentation Integrity (AHDI)
4230 Kiernan Avenue, Suite 130
Modesto, CA 95356
(800) 982-2182
Web site: http://www.ahdionline.org
Formerly known as the American Association for Medical
    Transcription, this organization provides certification
    and career resources for professionals involved in
    health care documentation. Its purpose is to protect the

integrity of patients' health information through continuous workforce development.

Canadian Association of Radiologists (CAR)
294 Albert Street, Suite 600
Ottawa, ON K1P 6E6
Canada
(613) 860-3111
Web site: http://www.car.ca
The national specialty society for radiologists in Canada, CAR is dedicated to maintaining the highest standards of care and promoting patient safety. The organization provides educational resources and a publication.

Canadian Society for Medical Laboratory Science (CSMLS)
33 Wellington Street North
Hamilton, ON L8R 1M7
Canada
(800) 263-8277
Web site: http://www.csmls.org
This organization provides certification of medical laboratory assistants and technologists. It also provides resources including medical news and a job bank.

Cardiovascular Credentialing International (CCI)
1500 Sunday Drive, Suite 102
Raleigh, NC 27607
(800) 325-0268
Web site: http://www.cci-online.org
CCI provides education and certification for cardiovascular technologists. Its Web site includes information

about its programs and events, as well as job listings.

National Council on the State Boards of Nursing (NCSBN)
111 East Wacker Drive, Suite 2900
Chicago, IL 60601-4277
(312) 525-3600
Web site: http://www.ncsbn.org
This organization provides licensing exams for various
    levels of nurses. It also provides a variety of publica-
    tions and online courses.

National Pharmacy Technician Association (NPTA)
P.O. Box 683148
Houston, TX 77268
(888) 247-8700
Web site: http://www.pharmacytechnician.org
NPTA provides certification for pharmacy technicians. It
    also offers a magazine and free newsletter, as well as
    information on jobs.

National Registry of Emergency Medical Technicians
    (NREMT)
Rocco V. Morando Building
6610 Busch Boulevard
Columbus, OH 43229
(614) 888-4484
Web site: http://www.nremt.org
This organization provides certification for EMTs at a
    variety of levels. Its Web site contains job listings.

Society of Diagnostic Medical Sonography (SDMS)
2745 Dallas Parkway, Suite 350
Plano, TX 75093-8730
(800) 229-9506
Web site: http://www.sdms.org
SDMS provides resources, including a scientific journal
and a newsletter, for ultrasound technologists.

Web Sites

Due to the changing nature of Internet links, Rosen
Publishing has developed an online list of Web sites
related to the subject of this book. This site is updated
regularly. Please use this link to access the list:

http://www.rosenlinks.com/HCC/Hosp

FOR FURTHER READING

Brezina, Corona. *Getting a Job in Health Care* (Job Basics: Getting the Job You Need). New York, NY: Rosen Publishing, 2014.

Christen, Carol, and Richard N. Bolles. *What Color Is Your Parachute? for Teens: Discovering Yourself and Your Future*. New York, NY: Ten Speed Press, 2010.

DeLaet, Roxann. *Introduction to Health Care & Careers*. Philadelphia, PA: Wolters Kluwer Health/Lippincott Williams & Wilkins, 2012.

Elsevier/Saunders. *Job Readiness for Health Professionals: Soft Skill Strategies for Success*. St. Louis, MO: Elsevier/Saunders, 2013.

Enelow, Wendy S., and Louise M. Kursmark. *Expert Résumés for Health Care Careers*. Indianapolis, IN: JIST Works, 2010.

Farr, Michael, and Laurence Shatkin. *300 Best Jobs Without a Four-Year Degree*. Indianapolis, IN: JIST Works, 2009.

Ferguson Publishing. *Careers in Focus: Medical Technicians and Technologists*. 5th ed. New York, NY: Ferguson, 2009.

Fitzpatrick, Joyce, and Emerson E. Ea (eds.). *201 Careers in Nursing*. New York, NY: Springer Publishing, 2011.

Griffin, Donald. *Hospitals: What They Are and How They Work*. Sudbury, MA: Jones & Bartlett, 2012.

Institute for Career Research. *Career as a Home Health Aide*. Chicago, IL: Institute for Career Research, 2012.

Kennedy, Joyce Lain. *Cover Letters for Dummies*. Hoboken, NJ: Wiley, 2009.

Kennedy, Joyce Lain. *Job Interviews for Dummies.* Hoboken, NJ: Wiley, 2011.

LearningExpress. *Becoming a Nurse.* New York, NY: LearningExpress, 2009.

Mumford, Colin, and Suvankar Pal. *Getting That Medical Job: Secrets for Success.* Hoboken, NJ: Wiley, 2011.

Prieto, Emily. *Home Health Care Provider: A Guide to Essential Skills.* New York, NY: Springer Publishing, 2008.

Reece, Richard. *Medicine* (Inside the Industry). Minneapolis, MN: Essential Library, 2011.

Routh, Kristiana Sue. *Professionalism in Medical Assisting.* Boston, MA: Pearson Education, 2014.

Strange, Cordelia. *Medical Technicians: Health-Care Support for the 21st Century* (New Careers for the 21st Century). Broomall, PA: Mason Crest Publishers, 2011.

Terry, Allison J. *The LPN-to-RN Bridge: Transitions to Advance Your Career.* Burlington, MA: Jones & Bartlett Learning, 2013.

BIBLIOGRAPHY

Colorado Department of Public Health and Environment. "EMS Provider Certification Frequently Asked Questions." Retrieved January 6, 2013 (http://www.colorado.gov).

Health Jobs Start Here. "Internships & Volunteering." Retrieved January 6, 2013 (http://www.health-jobsstarthere.com/resources/experience/find).

Health Jobs Start Here. "Nursing Aide/Nursing Attendant/Orderly." Retrieved January 6, 2013 (http://www.healthjobsstarthere.com/resources/job/Nursing-Aide-/-Nursing-Attendant-/-Orderly.html).

Health Jobs Start Here. "Scholarships & Financial Aid." Retrieved January 6, 2013 (http://www.health-jobsstarthere.com/resources/financial/scholarships).

Kintz, Jennifer. "What Being a Medical Assistant Is All About." AllAlliedHealthSchools.com. Retrieved March 7, 2013 (http://www.allalliedhealthschools.com/health-careers/medical-assisting/being-a-medical-assistant).

Morkes, Andrew, et al. *Hot Health Care Careers.* Chicago, IL: College & Career Press, 2011.

National Council of State Boards of Nursing. "NCLEX Examinations." 2013. Retrieved January 12, 2013 (https://www.ncsbn.org/nclex.htm).

New York City Fire Department. "EMT Saves Life of Man in Cardiac Arrest." NYC.gov. Retrieved January 19, 2013 (http://www.nyc.gov/html/fdny/html/events/2010/100710c.shtml).

U.S. Bureau of Labor Statistics. "EMTs and Paramedics." *Occupational Outlook Handbook,* March 29, 2012.

Retrieved April 9, 2013 (http://www.bls.gov/ooh /healthcare/emts-and-paramedics.htm).

U.S. Bureau of Labor Statistics. "Healthcare Occupations." *Occupational Outlook Handbook*, March 29, 2012. Retrieved January 19, 2013 (http://www.bls.gov/ooh/healthcare).

U.S. Census Bureau. "Expectation of Life at Birth, 1970 to 2008, and Projections, 2010 to 2020." *Statistical Abstract of the United States*, 2012. Retrieved January 19, 2012 (http://www.census.gov/compendia /statab/2012/tables/12s0104.pdf).

U.S. Department of Education. "Federal Supplemental Educational Opportunity Grant (FSEOG) Program." ED.gov, March 28, 2012. Retrieved January 8, 2013 (http://www2.ed.gov/programs/fseog/index.html).

U.S. Social Security Administration. "Social Security History: Life Expectancy for Social Security." SSA.gov, January 17, 2013. Retrieved January 19, 2013 (http://www.ssa.gov/history/lifeexpect.html).

Watson, Joe. *Where the Jobs Are Now: The Fastest-Growing Industries and How to Break into Them*. New York, NY: McGraw-Hill, 2010.

Wischnitzer, Saul, and Edith Wischnitzer. *Top 100 Health-Care Careers: Your Complete Guidebook to Training and Jobs in Allied Health, Nursing, Medicine, and More* (JIST Top Careers). 3rd ed. Indianapolis, IN: JIST Works, 2011.

INDEX

About the Author

Jeri Freedman has a B.A. from Harvard University. She has more than fifteen years' experience in sales and marketing for high-tech and medical products companies, including the Clinical Assays division of Baxter-Travenol. She is the author of more than thirty young adult nonfiction books, many published by Rosen Publishing, including *Careers in Emergency Medical Response Teams' Search and Rescue Units*; *Women in the Workplace: Wages, Respect, and Equal Rights*; *Being a Leader: Organizing and Inspiring a Group*; and *Careers in Pharmaceutical Sales*. Under the name Ellen Foxxe, she is the coauthor of two alternate history science-fiction novels.

Photo Credits

Cover (figure) Curt Pickens/E+/Getty Images; cover and interior pages (wheelchair) Ingram Publishing/Thinkstock; cover, back cover, p. 1 (background pattern) HunThomas/Shutterstock.com; pp. 4–5 (background) sfam photo/Shutterstock.com; p. 5 (inset) Scott Olson /Getty Images; pp. 10–11 John Moore/Getty Images; p. 13 Bloomberg/Getty Images; pp. 16–17, 22–23 Joe Raedle/Getty Images; pp. 27, 39, 42 The Washington Post/Getty Images; pp. 28–29 Orlando Sentinel/McClatchy-Tribune/Getty Images; p. 30 Tim Boyle/Getty Images; p. 31 Timothy A. Clary/AFP/Getty Images; p. 35 Mario Tama/Getty Images; p. 41 Matt Meadows /Peter Arnold/Getty Images; pp. 44, 52, 64–65 © AP Images; p. 48 Wavebreak Media/Thinkstock; p. 53 Kathryn Scott Osler /Denver Post/Getty Images; p. 58 Chris Hondros/Getty Images; p. 62 Hemera/Thinkstock.

Designer: Michael Moy; Editor: Andrea Sclarow Paskoff; Photo Researcher: Amy Feinberg